Walking in Faith:

A Tribute in Sonnets

Catherine McAuliffe, PhD

©2023 by Catherine McAuliffe

Published by Lititz Institute Publishing Division
PO Box 326, Lookout Mountain, TN 37350
www.lititzinstitute.org

Printed in the United States of America

First Edition January 2023

Library of Congress Cataloging-in-Publication Data

McAuliffe, Catherine

Walking in Faith: A Tribute in Sonnets   Catherine McAuliffe

            p.   cm.

        ISBN 978-1-7350067-1-0   (hardback)

1. Sonnets of Remembrance by Catherine McAuliffe
2. Photographs by Frank McAuliffe
3. Contemplative verse by Frank McAuliffe
4. A Tribute to Frank McAuliffe

Cover Photograph by Frank McAuliffe

This book relates the story of Two Loves walking together through a cherished spouse's illness and, ultimately, to his tragic death…
followed by a new spiritual journey for the bereaved spouse left behind.

But, more so, this book seeks to pay tribute to a life well-lived…

In loving memory of my cherished husband,
Francis J. McAuliffe
(Frank)

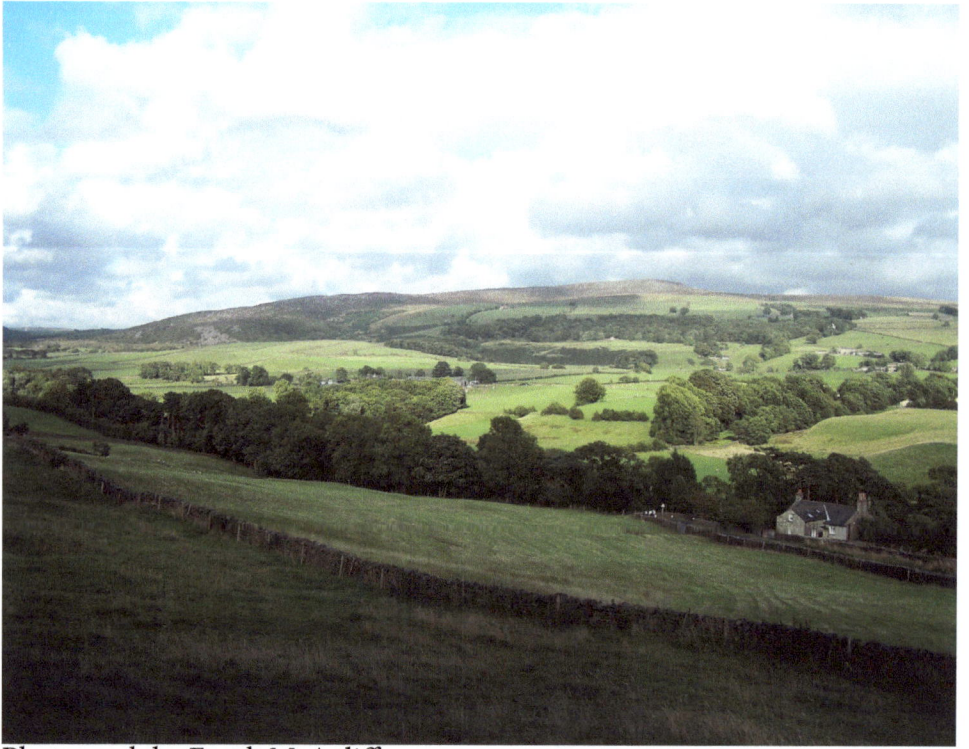

Photograph by Frank McAuliffe

ACKNOWLEDGEMENTS

I would like to begin by thanking Almighty God for continually blessing us each day with His Tender Care. I give particular thanksgiving for His having gifted my life so immeasurably with Darling Frank's deep love and devotion. He was a highly intelligent, talented person, as well, and thus I have been so immensely blessed. Frank is the inspiration for these sonnets.

I also wish to thank my dear friends, Dr. Bruce Williams, Maura Fox, and Reverend Edmund Nadolny, for having encouraged me to move forward with this project of love. I am truly grateful for your very kind support.

Additionally, I would like to thank everyone who gave Frank so much love and joy during his lifetime. He delighted in his family and friends, especially his three children, three step-children, and thirteen grandchildren. He was always enriched by each of you, as am I.

Blessings.

Catherine McAuliffe, PhD

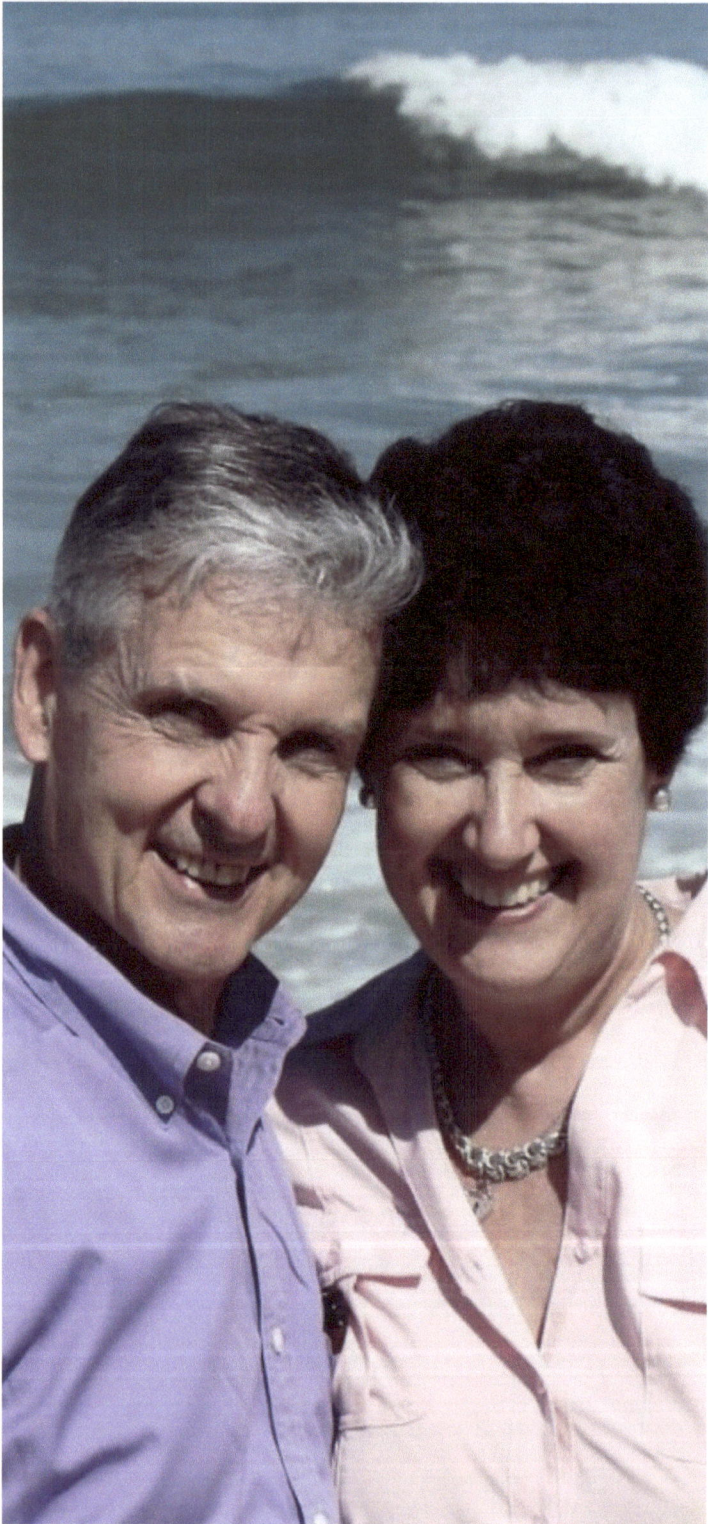

Frank and Catherine McAuliffe

FOREWORD

I have written this collection of sonnets as a tribute to my deceased husband, Francis J. McAuliffe. Frank was an utterly beautiful man who profoundly embraced a deep faith in God. He was the love of my life and soulmate for three decades.

My Love was also a gifted photographer who magnificently captured the beauty all around us. With a deep sense of pride, I have partnered a sampling of his photographs with these sonnets.

Engaging in sonnet-writing has served a twofold beneficial purpose: to grieve the loss of my husband and to memorialize his noble character. These sonnets are an expression of our joyful journeys, as well as our not-so-joyful walk with the devastation brought on by Alzheimer's Disease.

Frank suffered from the illness for more than five years, and I was privileged to have been his caregiver. But even during the darkest times, he still made every effort to care for me, too, as the devoted husband he always remained.

Frank's decline was heart-wrenching to witness, as he went from initially having the brilliant mind of the valedictorian of his prep school class, to becoming a brave veteran in that brutal war against his mental and bodily functioning.

Throughout the journey, we both turned to God, as was our practice. Ultimately, God's Grace sustained the two of us then, as it does me, now.

These sonnets relate our journey:
from the point of having received his diagnosis;
through the years of active Alzheimer's;
to his tragic death;
and to my subsequent grief and ongoing spiritual healing.
The last sonnets are a final tribute to this wonderful man.

This is a love story.

A sonnet is a poem that has fourteen lines, ten beats each, with a rhyme scheme of: ababcdcdefefgg.

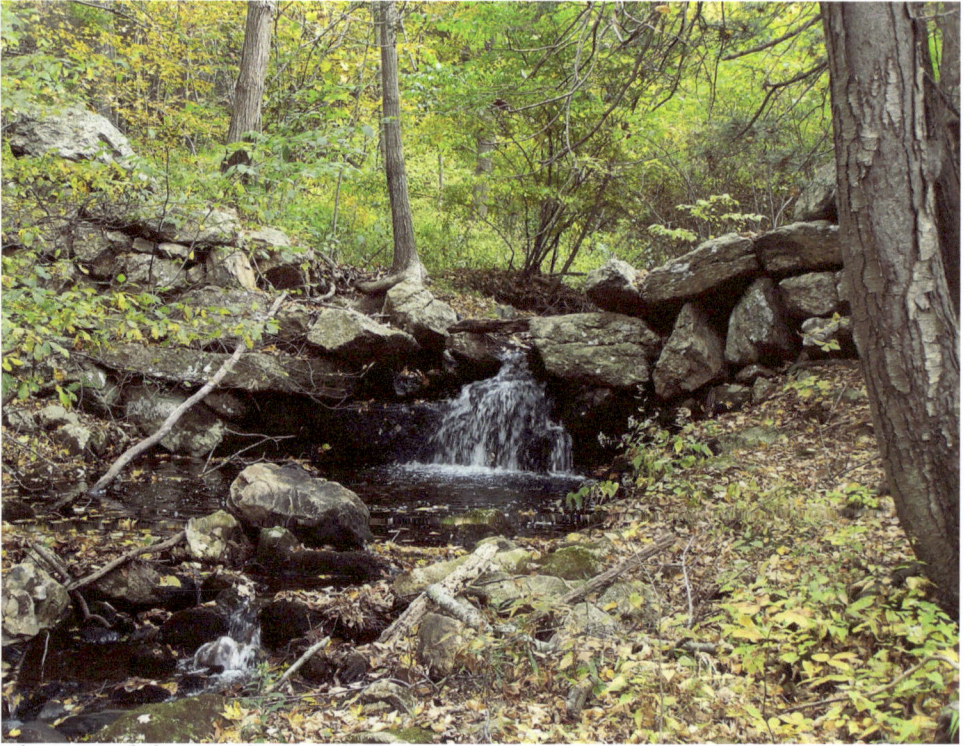

Photograph by Frank McAuliffe

Table of Contents

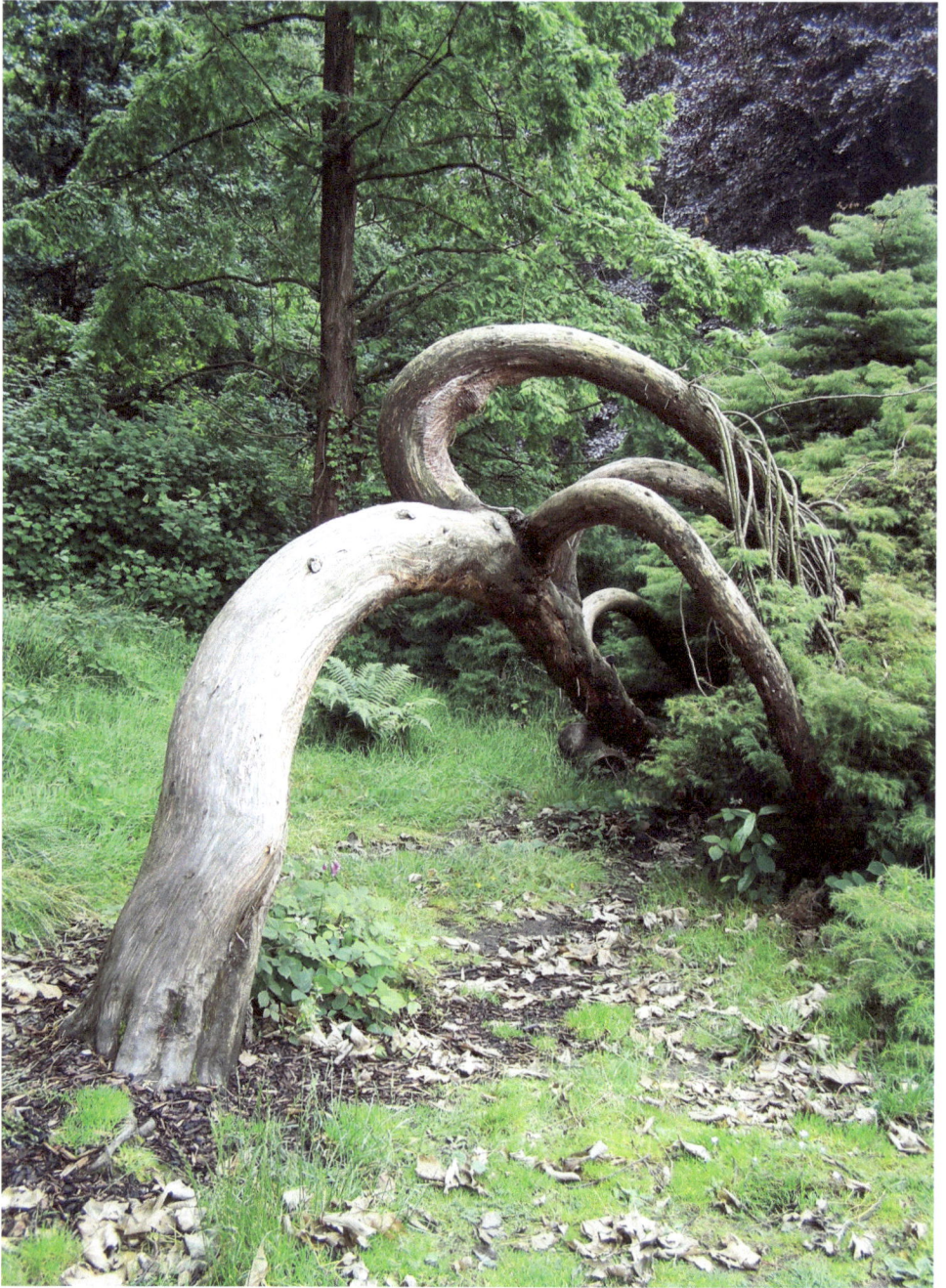

Photograph by Frank McAuliffe

The News

The two of us went together that day

To My Love's knee replacement surgery.

He had great difficulty in the way

He came out of his anesthesia. He

Was agitated, slow to awaken

And was confused, with some memory loss.

Months later, a CT scan had us shaken…

His brain had shrunken: Our personal cross.

Then his amyloids were found: Alzheimer's.

This was in his genes, but began to show

Quite suddenly. These events were just blurs…

Our journey began. We were worried so

And thought we'd not know happiness again…

But Our Lord would strengthen us through the pain.

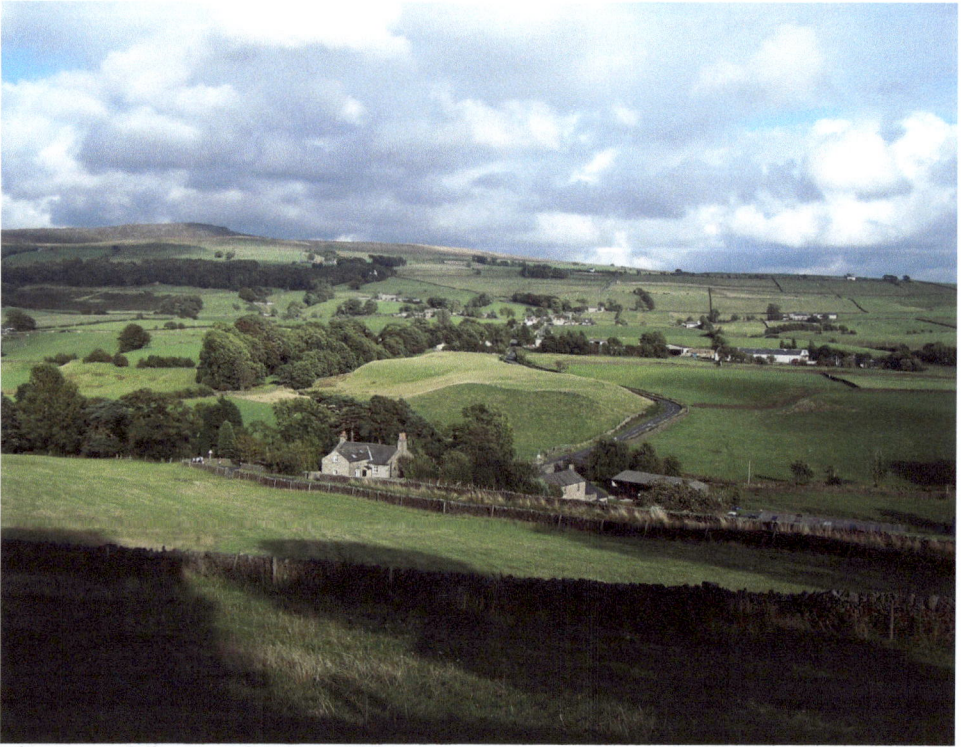

Photograph by Frank McAuliffe

We Shall Both Walk in Faith and Unity

As we begin each new day, Our God is

Continually blessing our lives, near

Us, every step of the way; for this

Is His Promise, and so we should not fear.

His Faithfulness and Mercy uphold us,

As we are caressed in His Tender Care.

He calms our souls through this journey, and thus,

We trust in Him, for He is truly there,

With us through this gray storm, lighting our way.

Challenges may blur our focus on Him,

If we were to let them. But we must lay

Every dark burden that we face in

His Strong Arms, to be strengthened and set free.

We shall both walk in faith and unity.

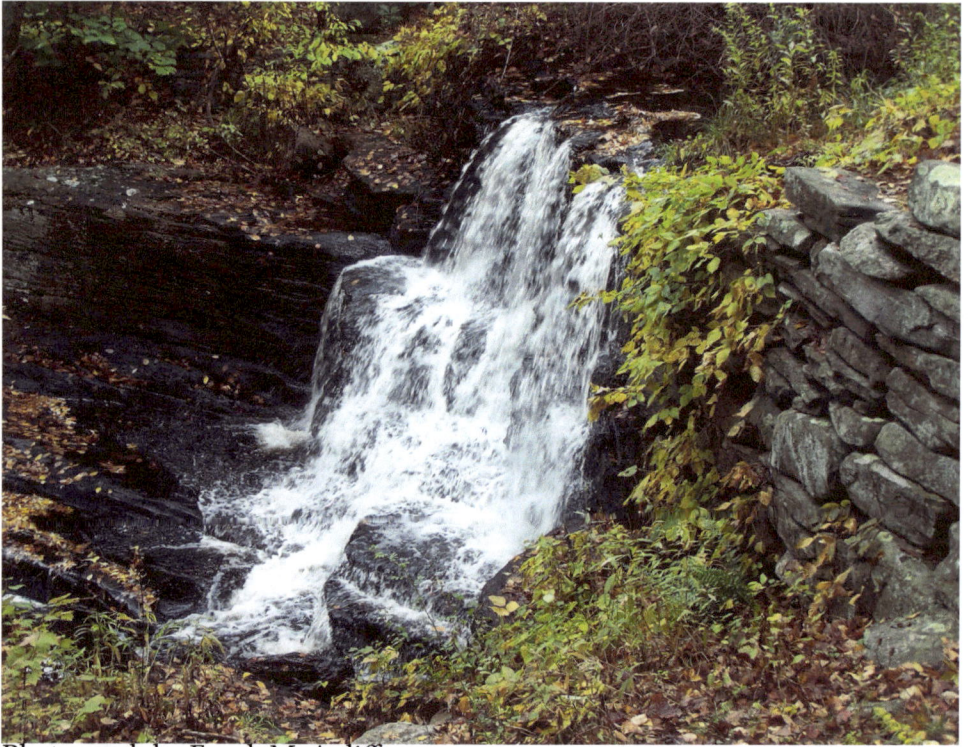

Photograph by Frank McAuliffe

Your Bravery Brings Me Such Pride

There are many types of brave souls I've met,

But, Sweet Love, you rank among the most brave.

You remain upbeat and kind and don't let

This dark illness impact how you behave.

You smile often and extend so much love,

Beyond the call of duty, ev'ry day.

To us, you're an angel sent from above,

Who richly blesses us in ev'ry way.

You have suffered so much with this disease,

And yet with such grace, you carry your cross.

We ask that Our Lord may comfort you please,

And give you His Strength, as you face such loss.

Partners on this journey, I'm by your side;

Your brav'ry, My Treasure, brings me such pride.

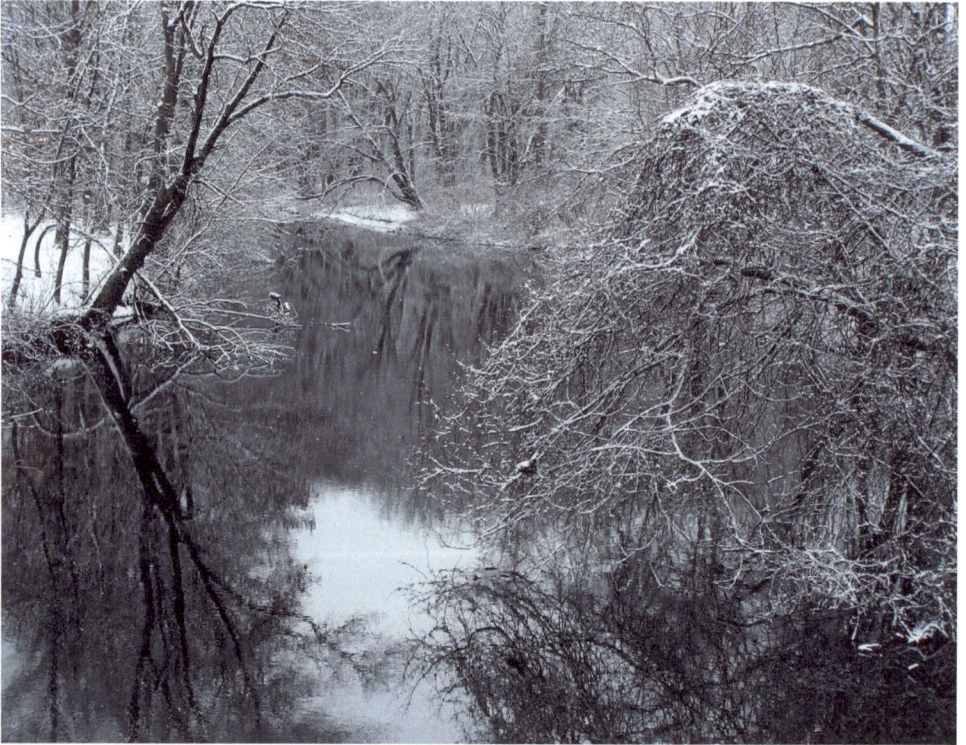

Photograph by Frank McAuliffe

We Wait Upon Your Perfect Plan

We're walking in faith... and gratitude, too,

For each gift You send us along our way.

Lord, Your Tender Care enfolds us; may You

Please grant My Love Divine Healing today?

As his caregiver, I can't untangle

His dementia and give him new options,

As he bravely fights that which will strangle

His mental and his bodily functions.

True clarity, once present, has now waned,

Yet dignity shines in this precious man.

We're steadfast in prayer, and thus sustained,

While we wait, Lord, upon Your Perfect Plan.

Only in You shall we find lasting hope,

As You bless us both, and help us to cope.

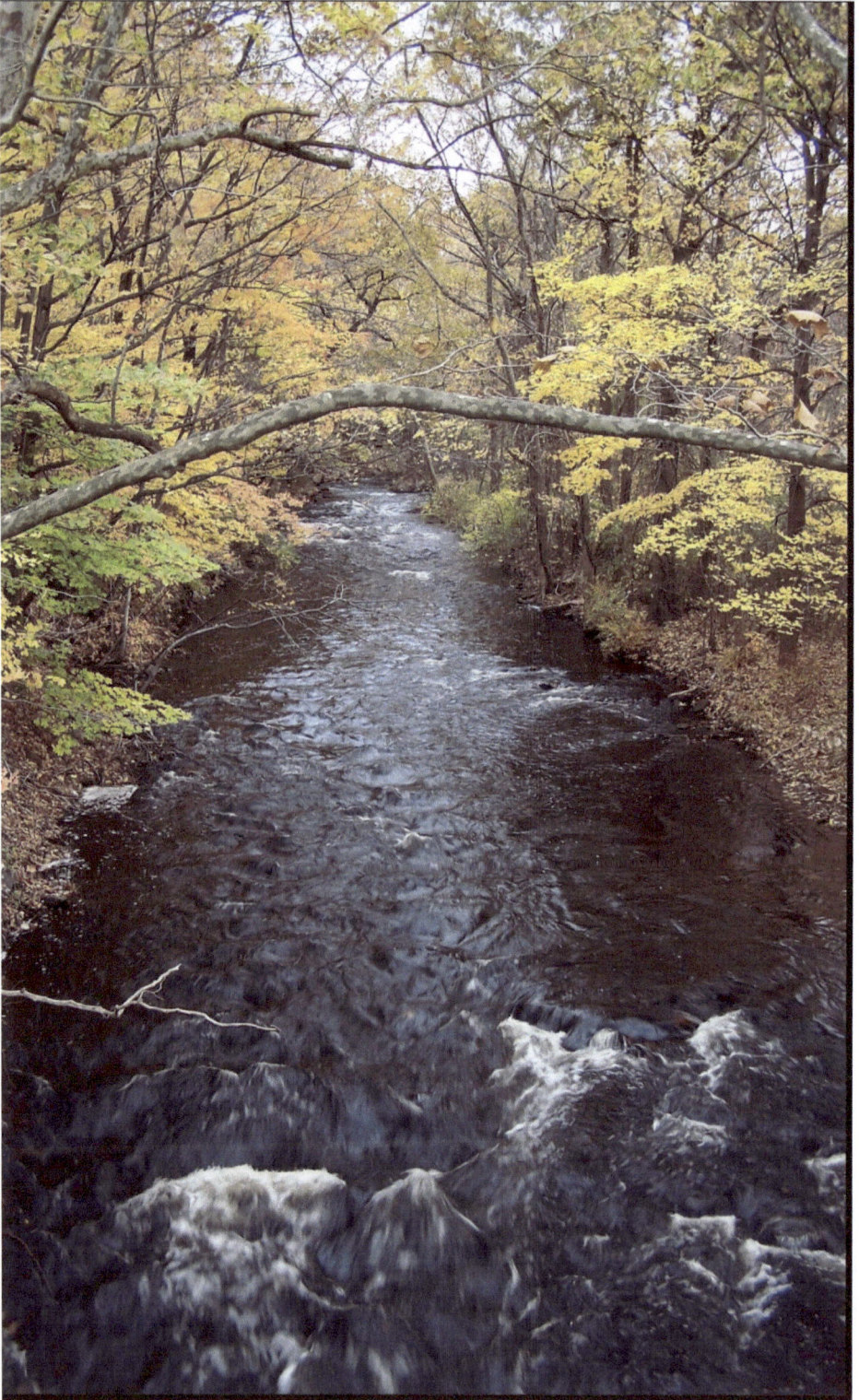

Photograph by Frank McAuliffe

Caregivers

During this long journey that we travel,

There are a special few who deeply know

The true challenges of caregivers well.

These precious gems understand just how low

I may find myself as I give my all,

And my all is not enough to hold back

The insidious nature of death's call.

How horrific is the raging attack,

As this illness, so brutally unkind,

Robs with fury the function and essence

Of My Cherished Love's once capable mind.

But I am not alone, I know, and hence,

How tremendously I appreciate

Other dear caregivers who share this fate.

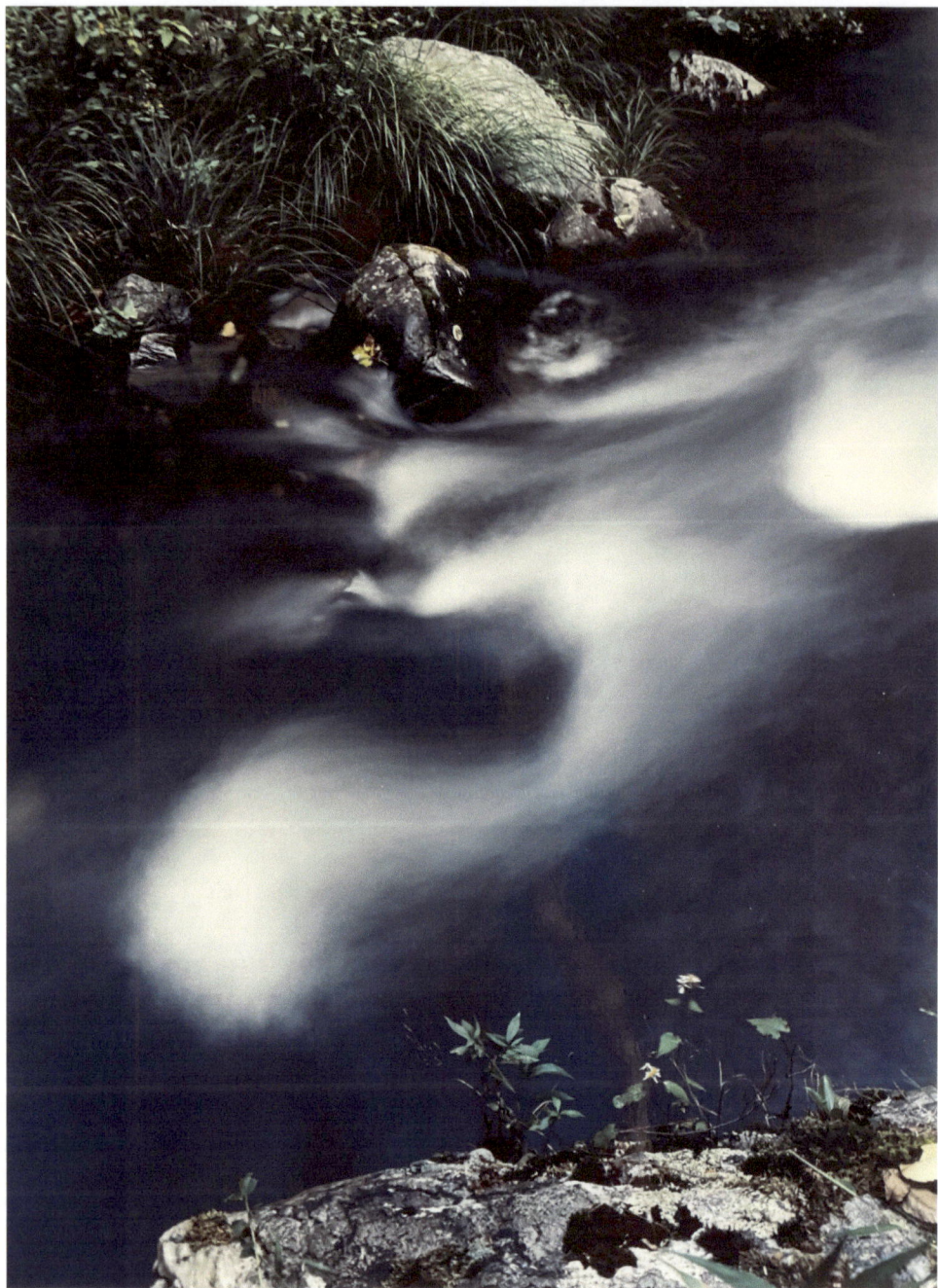
Photograph by Frank McAuliffe

This I Promise

You are My Love, My Dearest, forever,

For it's you I hold, ever close to me.

What joy it is to share days we treasure,

Knowing God alone knows just what will be.

But what pain I feel as you slip away

From me, right before my eyes, more and more.

This thief does not stop stealing you each day,

Taking those parts of you that I adore.

How thankful I am for glimmers of gold…

Remnants remaining of my true lover.

As I cherish joyful moments we hold,

I guard against darkness that may hover.

This passion that's ours will never grow cold:

This I promise… from the depths of my soul!

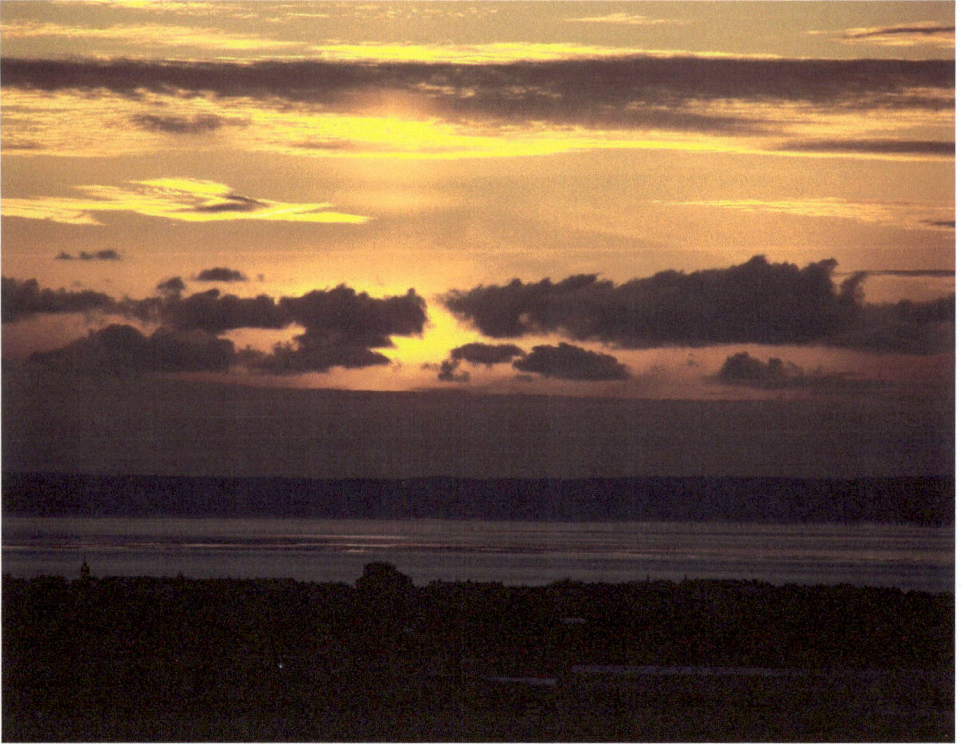

Photograph by Frank McAuliffe

That Fateful Night: Part I

That fateful night when we turned in to bed,

My Darling began to wildly convulse:

A true nightmare… I thought he may be dead…

But no, thank God, there seemed to be a pulse.

I shook him firmly giv'n the circumstance,

And called out his name. He came back to me!

At the same time, I dialed the ambulance.

Next Stop: The E.R. - They worked desp'rately.

He passed once, but he returned, trying so

To stay with us. But then, devastation:

He left this earthly realm… oh no, no, no.

It was too soon. I felt desperation

And pain to have lost the love of my life…

It was as if I'd been stabbed with a knife.

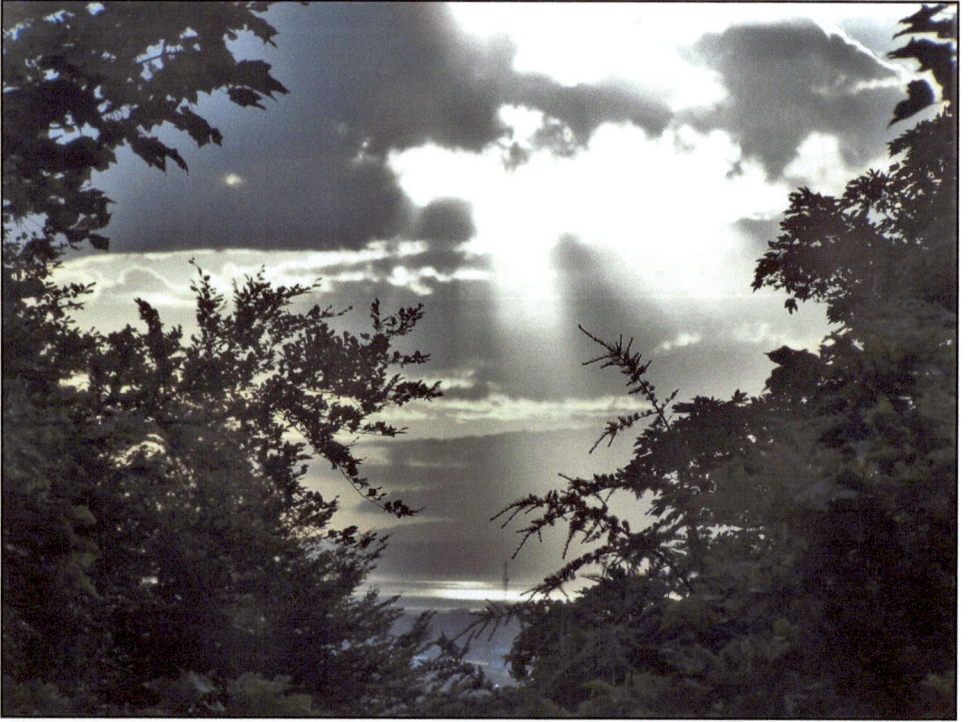

Photograph by Frank McAuliffe

That Fateful Night: Part II

That night, I felt such horror with the news;

This was truly my earthly heart's response.

My Darling was not with me… No excuse

Could help me be reconciled to this loss.

Then my spiritual heart began to tell

The truth: God had taken My Sweet Love Home.

He had lived his whole life on earth to dwell

With Our Lord for all the ages to come.

His second birth had won him God's Mercy.

I felt peace that he was with his Lord… not

On a fateful night, but one of glory.

It was time to gain the reward he'd sought.

My Dearest Love is now out of his pain,

Never to know any suff'ring again.

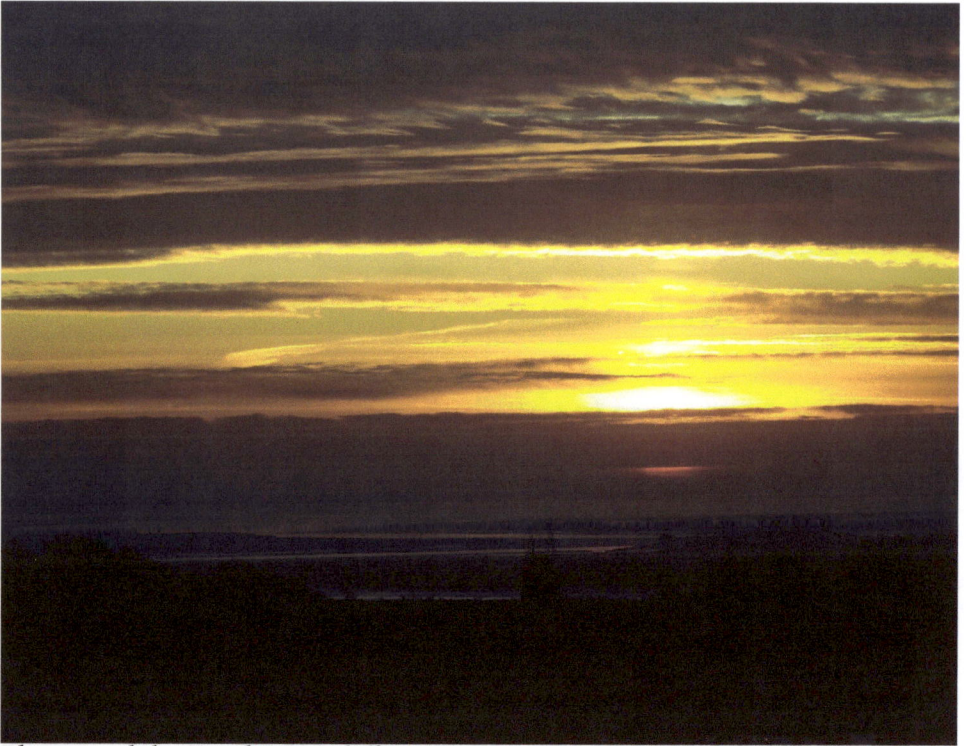

Photograph by Frank McAuliffe

I'll Hold You Again

Time spent with you was filled with such beauty.

What pleasure I knew being by your side!

Your soul was filled with rarest purity,

And, in ev'ry way, you brought me true pride.

Throughout the months and years and then decades,

Our love grew in ways so unimagined.

Joy was embellished by your serenades

Of those sweet romantic songs! Ah… but then…

We faced the grip of that dreaded disease

That took your life, but not our love that binds.

Separated, for now, are our bodies,

But not our spirits. Hope ever reminds

Me, that when reaching the everlasting,

I'll hold you again, My Treasured Darling!

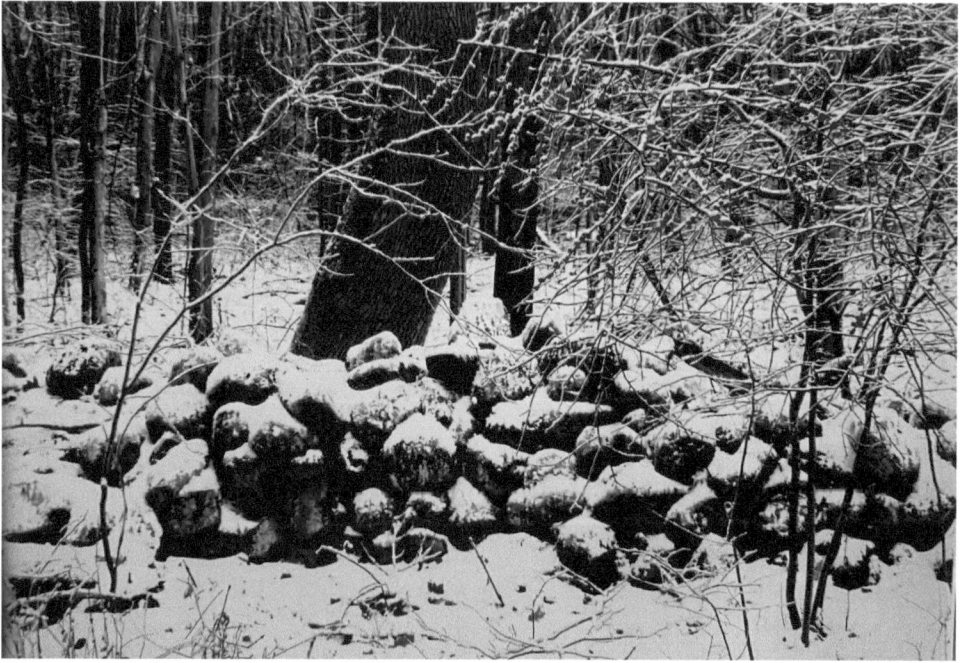
Photograph by Frank McAuliffe

In Life's Winter Season

The winter of our lives had come our way,

Bringing new challenges for us to face;

But how we loved each other ev'ry day,

And, thus, treasured each sweet moment's embrace.

Together, we journeyed through your illness,

Not knowing just where it may one day lead;

Yet, we found comfort amidst the darkness,

As God sent us strength for every need.

Wisdom teaches that pain is halved when shared;

Truly, we found this to be so for us.

We walked in love's realm, beautifully paired,

While making mem'ries that are so precious!

Yes, in life's winter season, love's pleasure

Still bloomed, Dear… with beauty, beyond measure…

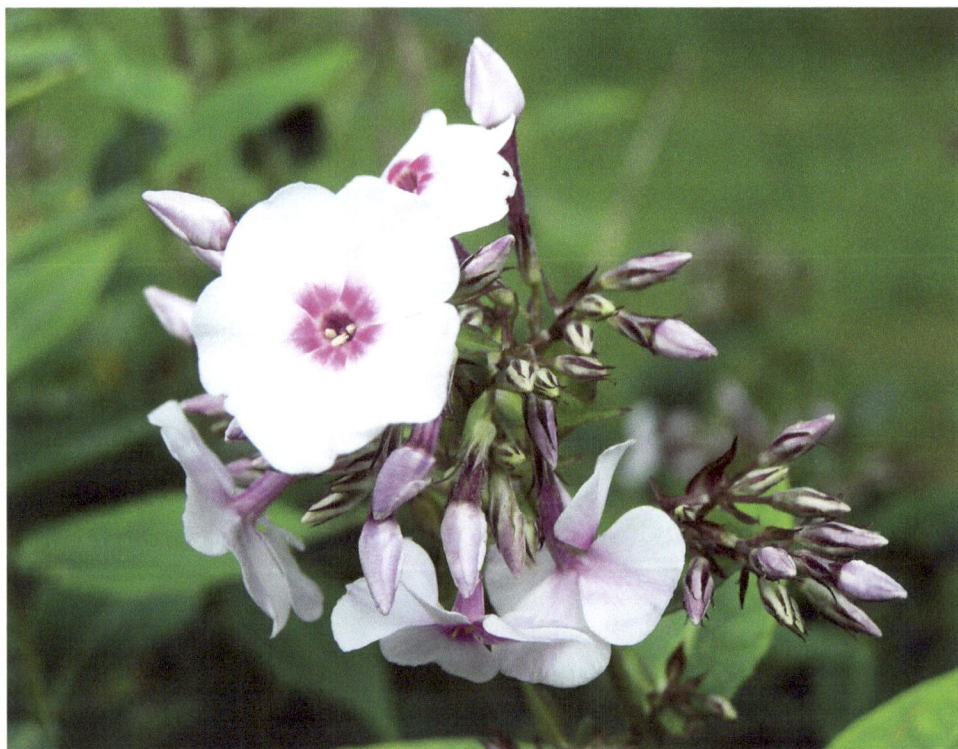

Photograph by Frank McAuliffe

Always in My Heart

My Precious Love, I long for you to be

Right here next to me, like when all was fine.

As we shared our love so very deeply,

What joy was ours, Dearest Husband of Mine!

You enriched my life more than you can know,

And, truly, ev'ry day you made me beam.

Your kind and chivalrous ways charmed me so!

You've been the beautiful man of my dreams,

And it's those mem'ries that I hold onto.

Thoughts of happy times are worth more than gold!

These days, peace can be mine, knowing that you

Now have God's Presence ever to behold.

Till we meet again, Dear, we're not apart,

For I'll keep our love always in my heart.

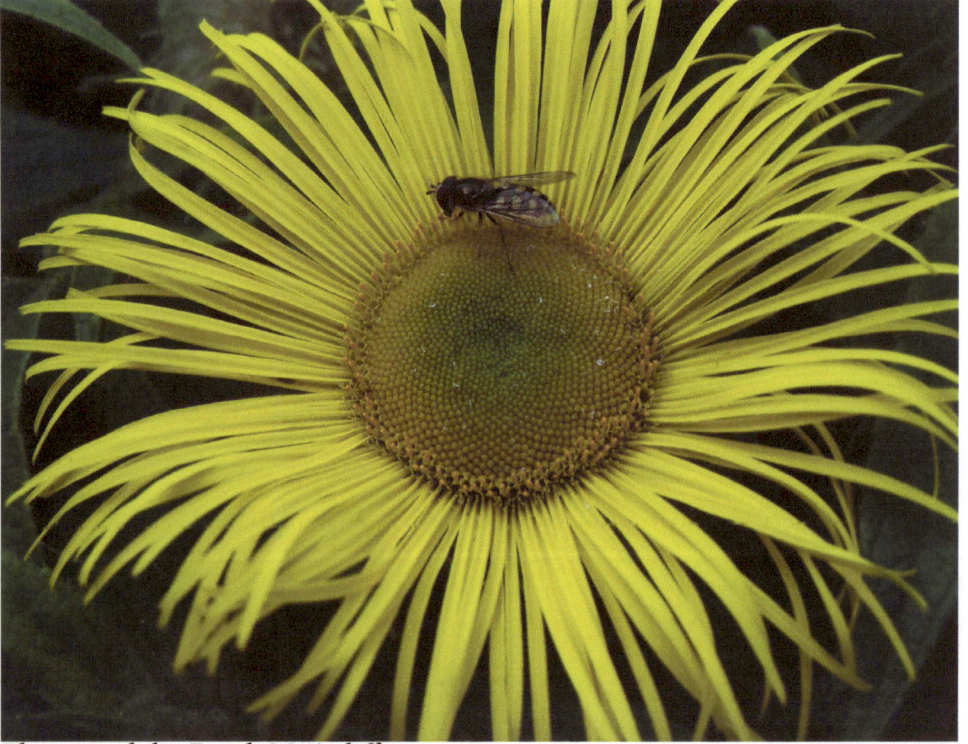

Photograph by Frank McAuliffe

Just One More Day

I had the dearest thoughts of you anew,

Today as I strolled down a garden path.

A daydream began to form about you:

As I envisioned your wonderful laugh,

You began to walk along by my side,

Loving this place with perfume in the air!

And as I held your arm, I felt such pride

With My Darling here, once again… a pair,

Going back in time for just one more day.

How we beamed as we felt that special joy,

Basking in love in our own precious way.

But, alas, you're not here, though I enjoy

Sav'ring an imagined outing's pleasure

With the precious man I'll always treasure.

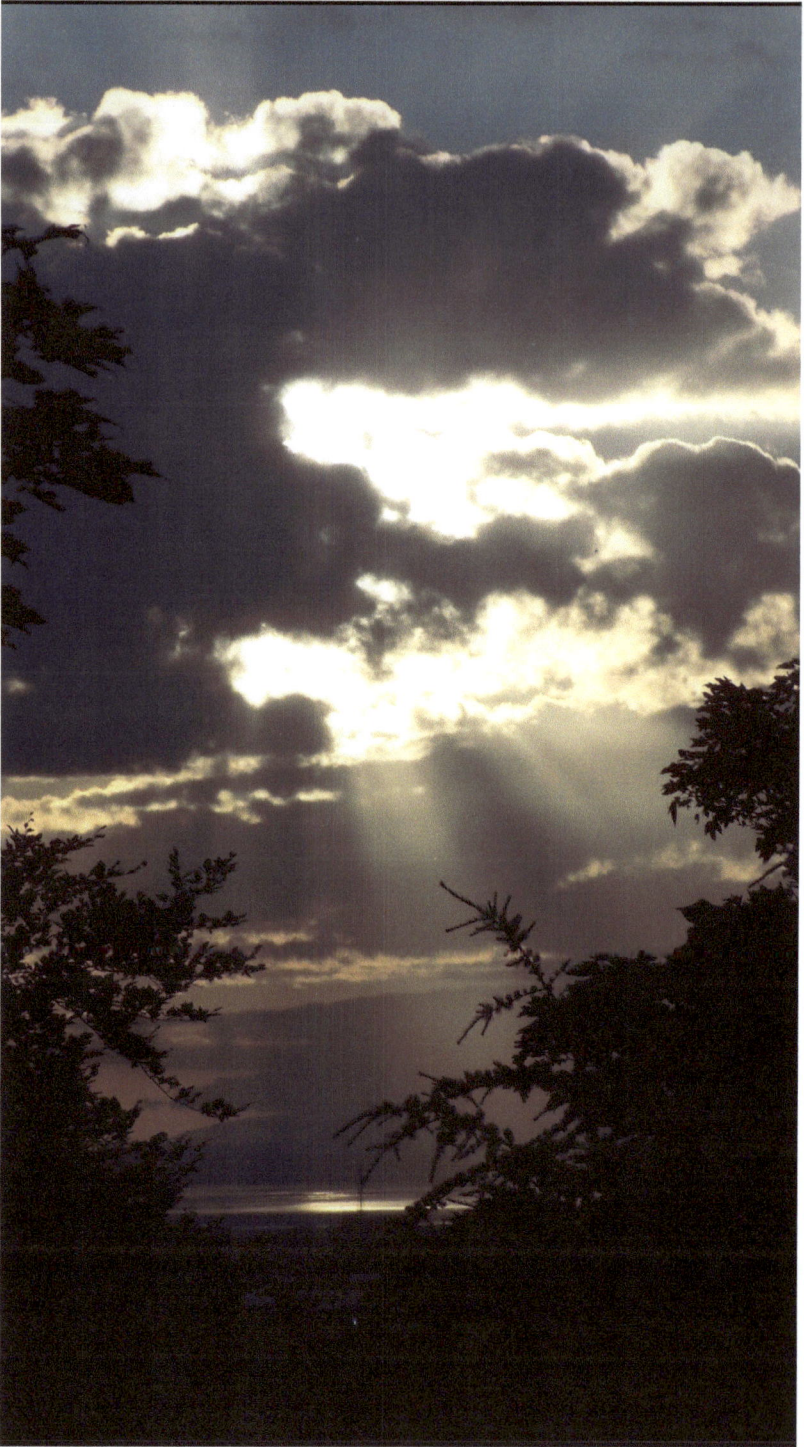

Photograph by Frank McAuliffe

How Wondrous It Will Be

Darling Love, as I start to doze tonight,

I sense you're near me, but then remember

That Our Dear Lord took you into His Light

Where peace will be yours forever after.

You no longer know the plight of illness,

Nor feel that confusion as it gripped you

For more than five years, taking the essence

Of your mind, yes, your very being, too.

You've been freed now to join the saints above,

And rejoice ever in God's Joy and Grace!

How I will always treasure your soul's love,

As I deeply cherish each sweet embrace.

But, oh how much more wondrous it will be

When we shall meet again in ecstasy!

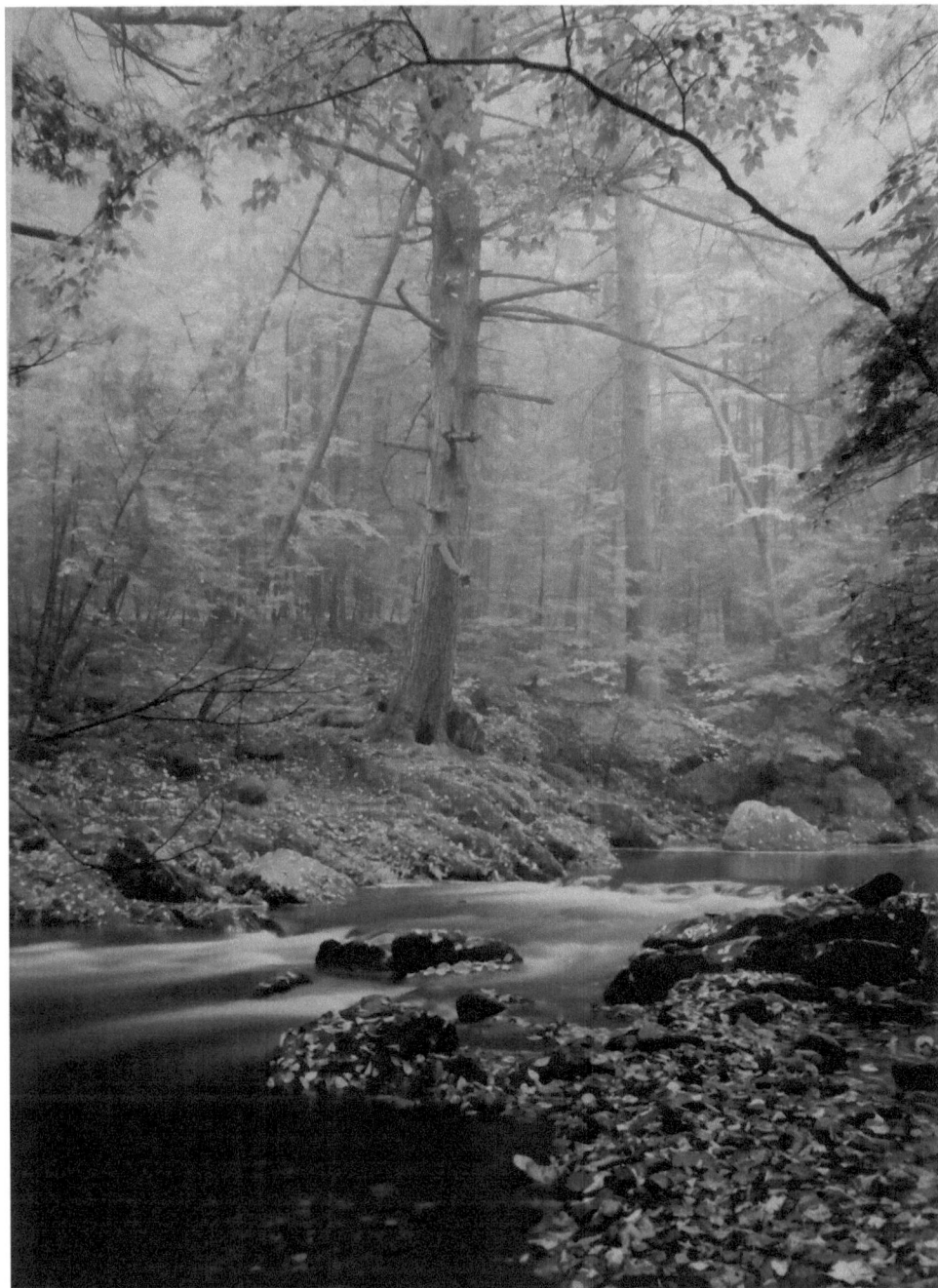

Photograph by Frank McAuliffe

My Soul is Tenderly Blessed

Although I live alone now since you've passed,

I know Our Loving Lord renews my soul.

He's my Comforter, if I miss the past,

And long for days with happiness untold.

But unhelpful thoughts I cannot dwell on,

For I wish to follow in God's way. In

Him, I am sustained, as I lay upon

His Caring Heart, concerns from deep within.

The Transforming Love of God anoints me,

As my soul's blessed in such a tender way…

Gently… in peaceful waters… endlessly…

So, Dear, I want you to know that each day,

As I learn to cope with your loss, Sweet Love,

My soul is tenderly blessed from above.

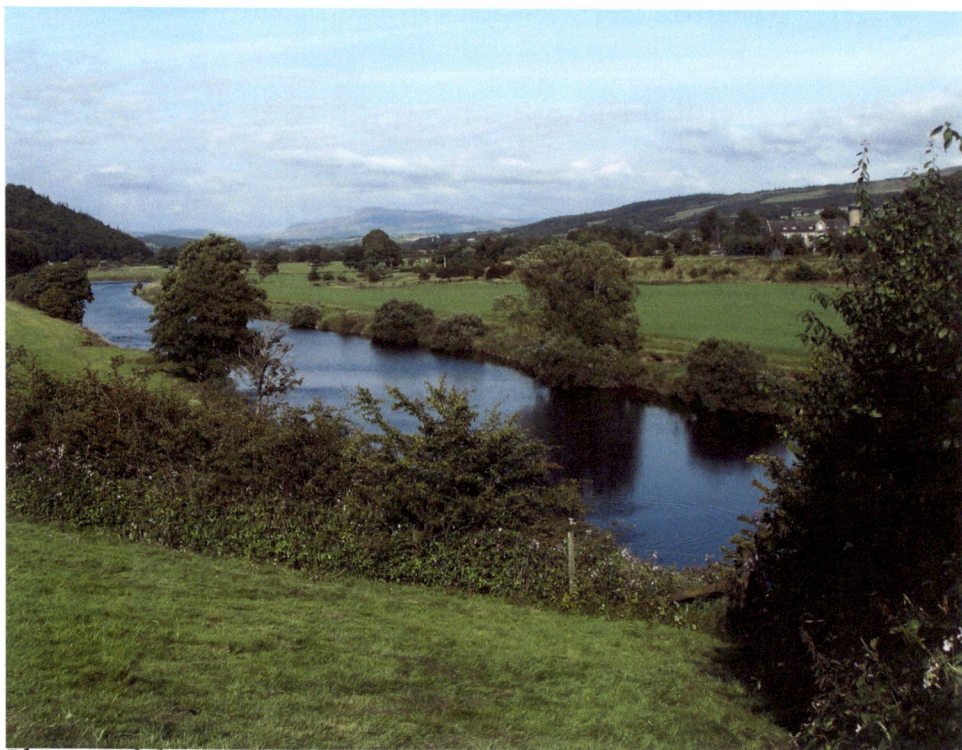

Photograph by Frank McAuliffe

A Widow's Prayer

I come before You, Lord, with gratitude

For all Your many blessings that are mine.

As I praise You, I know with certitude

That You hear me with Your Mercy Divine.

Knowing this won'drous truth, should I have fears,

Or hold onto the pain of a widow?

No… You protect me, even amidst tears,

So sadness may never fester and grow.

Your Grace is sufficient, this I profess,

And boast of Your Pow'r, which rests on my soul.

Thus, fully trusting in Your Faithfulness,

This widow is being healed and consoled.

Bathing me in Your Love, You'll walk with me

Now, on earth… and throughout eternity.

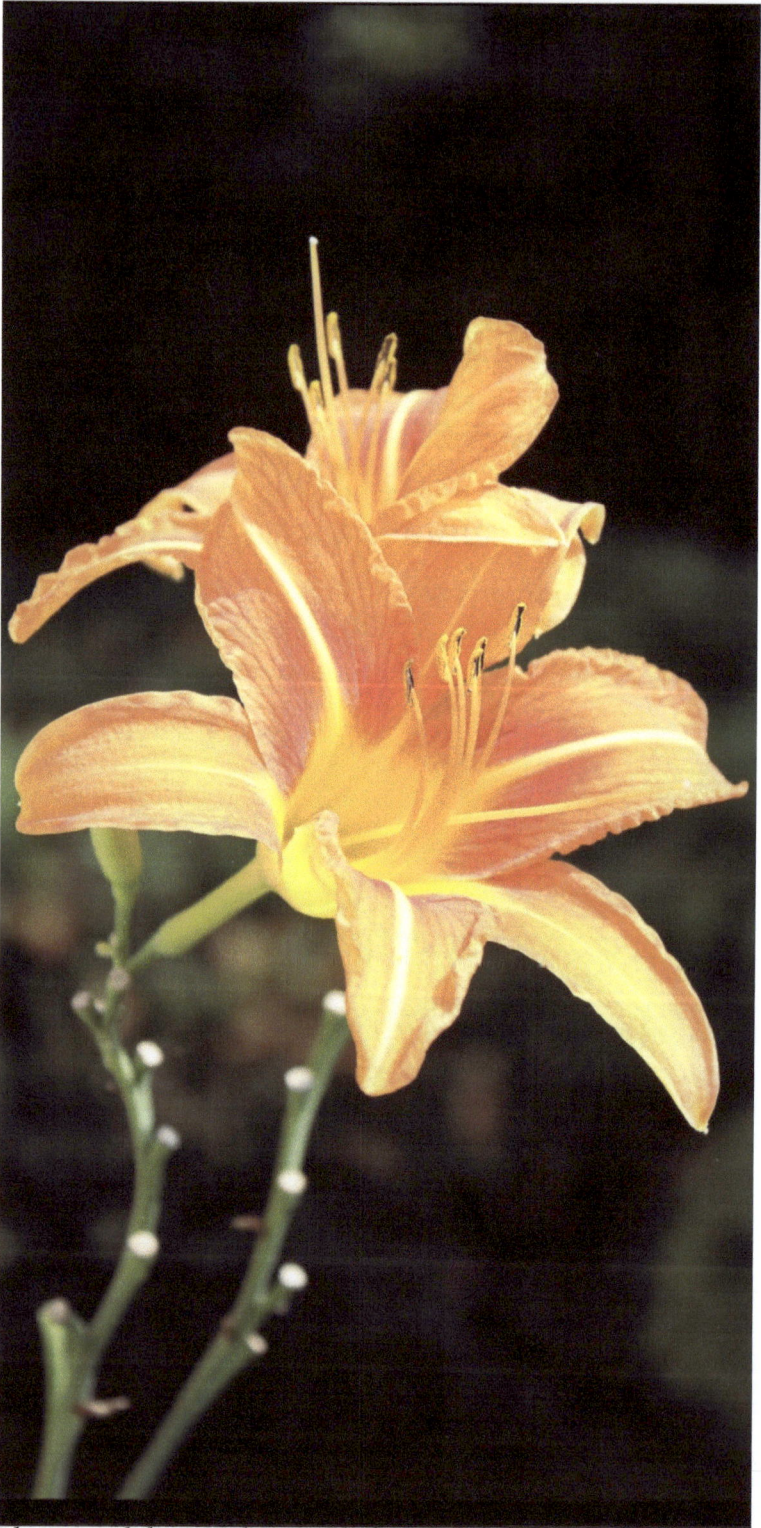

Photograph by Frank McAuliffe

A Gift of Great Beauty

My Dearest Love, through our journeys each day,

We've been blessed and challenged by many things.

A range of emotions have come our way,

But, united, we have met what life brings.

Finding love as soul-mates, we've shared such bliss,

And formed such a bond as the best of friends.

Those decades of pure joy, I dearly miss;

But I am thankful our love never ends.

Later, we met with dark trials brought on by

That dreaded disease that ended your days,

But with such grace, you carried your cross; I

Will always cherish all your noble ways!

God has giv'n us a gift of great beauty:

Ours has been such a treasured love story!

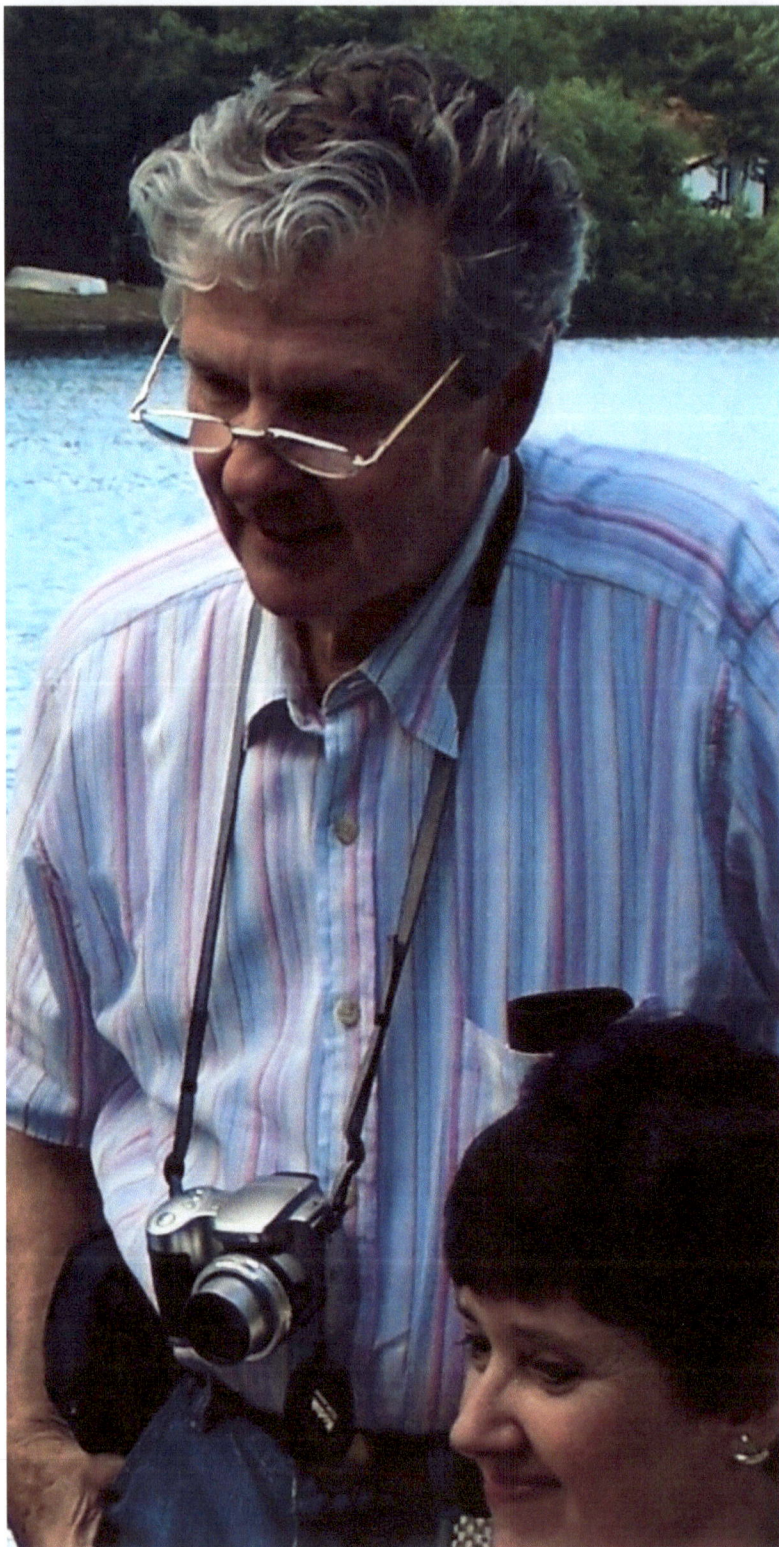
Photographer, Frank McAuliffe, with his camera

46

What Joy You Have Given

What talents you've always had, My Darling.

You began your career in radio

And t.v. production and broadcasting.

Twenty years, and then it was time to go

Into teaching college photography.

Students loved you and got their B.F.A.'s.

As you photographed professionally,

You captured products, nature, wedding days…

While thirty five years as a professor,

And thirty years, too, at the post offices.

Through the decades, your voice, as well, did soar

At fine restaurants and church services.

Remaining humble, as your gifts have shone,

What joy you have given to all you've known!

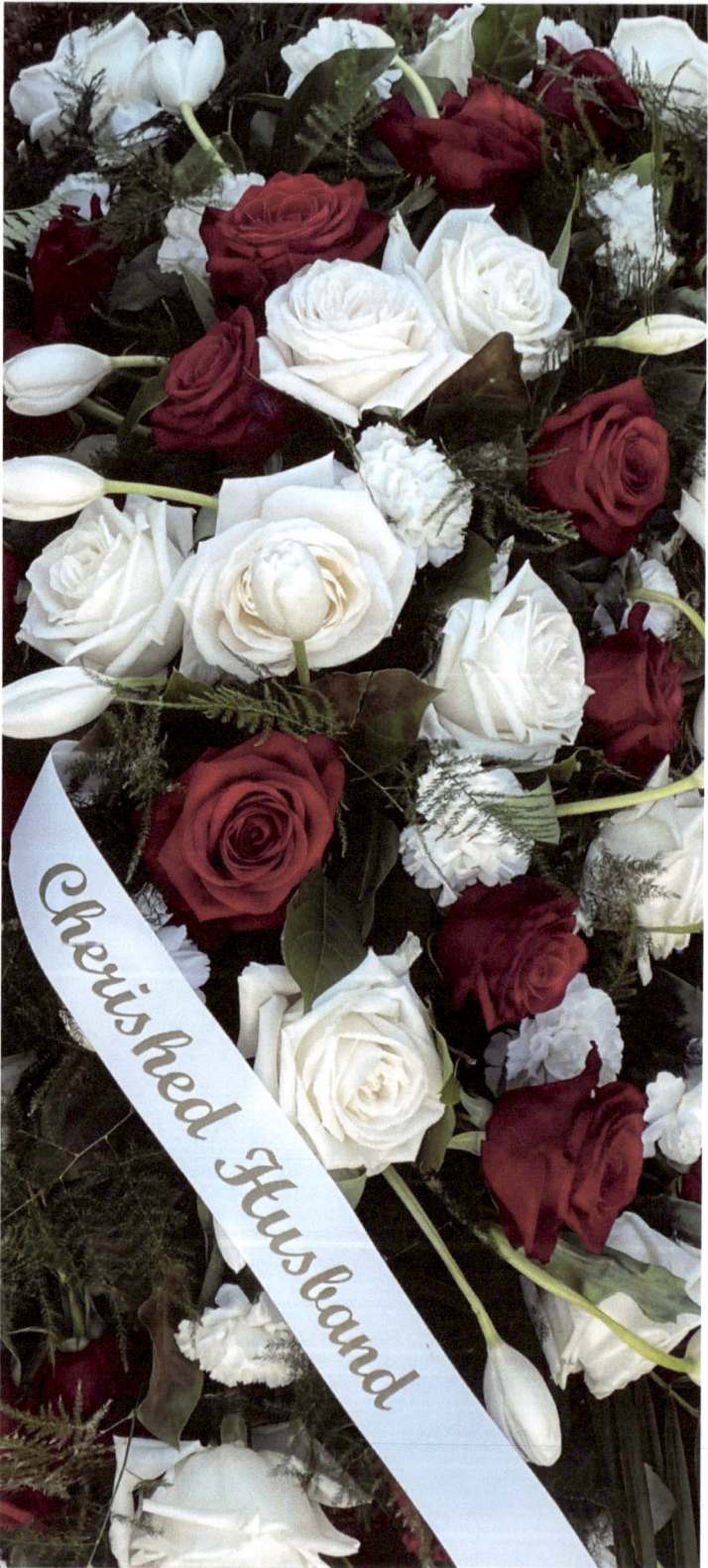

I Pay Tribute to Your Life Well-Lived

How could I ever say good bye to you

As loves of our lives and very best friends?

The truth is, I will not and don't have to.

Love goes beyond the grave and never ends.

As I pay tribute to your life well-lived,

I'm truly beaming with great pride in you.

In blissful times and those we just "survived",

You've been ever a fount of love so true,

As your immense faith in God shone daily.

Your talents, intelligence, and kindness

Have enriched so many eternally.

Dear, you're cherished for your great giftedness …

And the utter joy you've shared for all time!

I'LL THANK YOU ALWAYS …
TREASURED LOVE OF MINE!

Frank's Contemplative Verse and Photograph

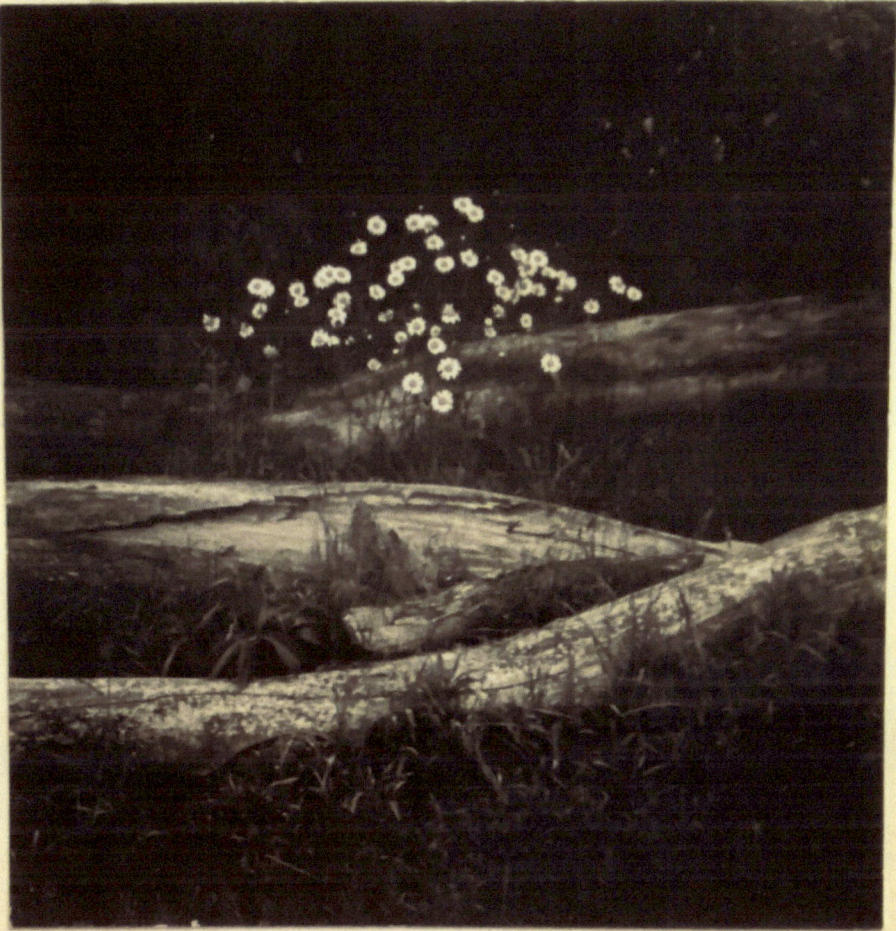

JUST AS NEW BLOSSOMS
EMERGE IN THE SHADOW
OF THE FALLEN TREE.

So THE NEW YEAR
BRINGS FORTH FRESH HOPE
FROM THE SHADOW OF THE OLD.
Frank McAuliffe

In Loving Memory of Francis J. McAuliffe

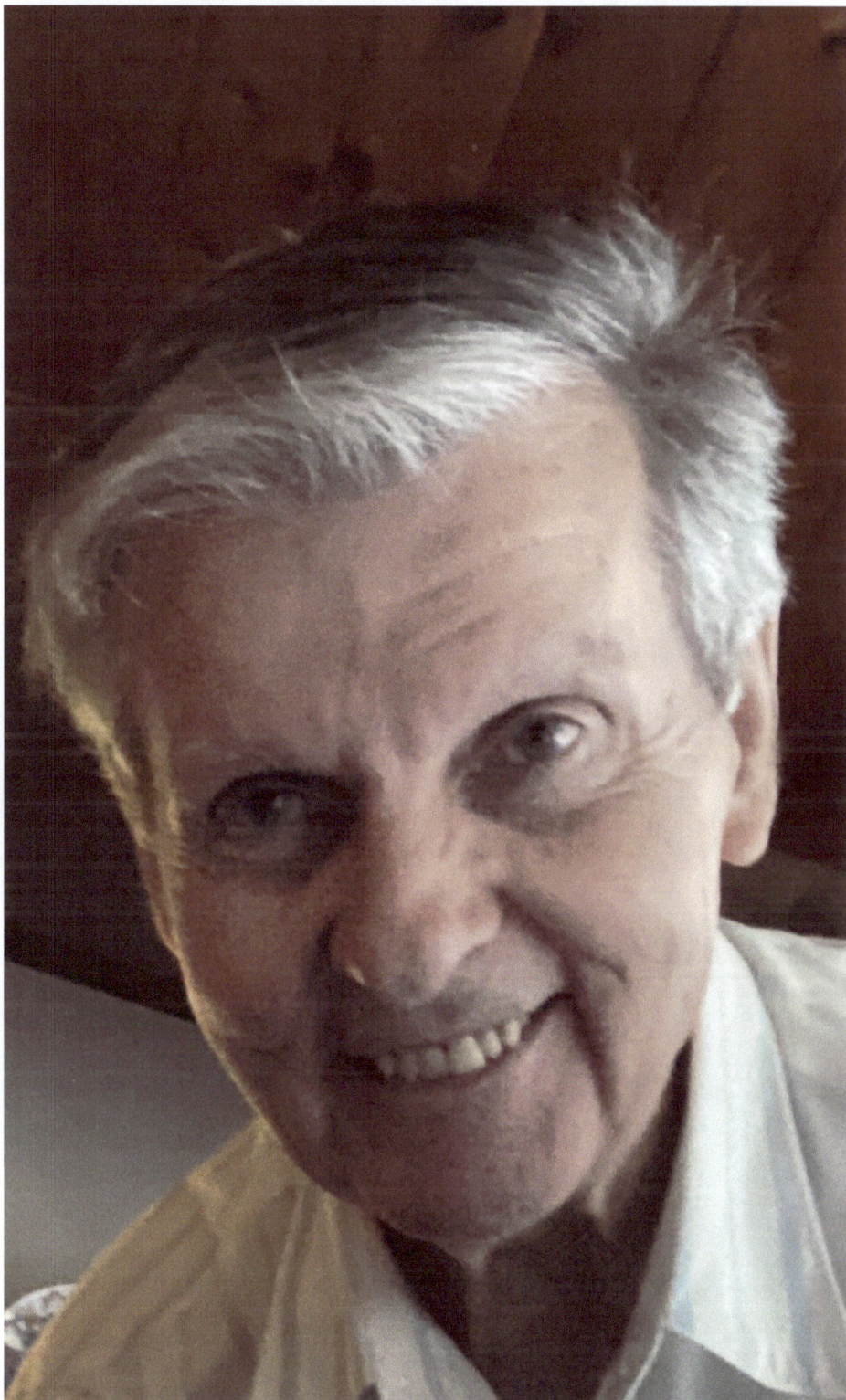

About the Author

Catherine McAuliffe, PhD, has served in the field of counseling for thirty five years and is presently a mental health therapist in private practice. In earlier years, she enjoyed her position as a college psychology professor for about a decade. She began her career as an elementary school teacher. More recently, she created and implemented a research-based Teacher S.U.P.P.O.R.T. Model to empower teachers.

Catherine's other life ventures have included singing and playing keyboard and guitar for three decades at weddings, funerals, and worship services. Her beloved husband, Frank, joined her as a vocalist during most of those years. Additionally, she has composed twenty sacred songs which have been sung by church choirs in her native Connecticut.

While Catherine was studying for her doctorate in England, she was accompanied by Frank, who was a professional photographer. Most of the photographs in this book were taken by him during their visits to the United Kingdom.

Catherine has written this book of sonnets as a tribute to her deceased husband, Frank, who was the love of her life for thirty years. Their lives have been blessed and enriched by their six children and thirteen grandchildren.

JUMP FOR JORDAN

DONNA ABELA

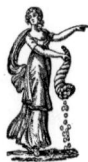

Currency Press,
Sydney

CURRENCY PLAYS

First published in 2014
by Currency Press Pty Ltd,
PO Box 2287, Strawberry Hills, NSW, 2012, Australia
enquiries@currency.com.au
www.currency.com.au

in association with Griffin Theatre Company

This revised edition first published in 2017 by Currency Press.

Cataloguing-in-Publication data for this title is available from the National Library of Australia website: www.nla.gov.au

Typeset by Dean Nottle for Currency Press.
Cover design by Alissa Dinallo for Currency Press.
Cover shows Al Khazneh at Petra, Jordan. Photo by Oleg Znamenskiy [Shutterstock].